MONTH ▴ OF ▴ MEALS ▴ 2
A ▴ MENU ▴ PLANNER

Published by the American Diabetes Association

ISBN 0-945448-15-5

TABLE OF CONTENTS

ACKNOWLEDGEMENTS

This publication has been created by a committee of the Council on Nutritional Science and Metabolism of the American Diabetes Association (ADA). The committee included Marion Franz, M.S., R.D., Nancy Cooper, R.D., Lois Babione, M.S., R.D., Anne Daly, M.S., R.D., and Robin Williams, M.A., R.D. Staff members of the ADA National Center also contributed to this publication, in particular Mary T. Linden, Kim Fawcett, Donald Jewler, and Susan H. Coughlin.

The recipes in *Month of Meals 2* come from several sources. We wish to acknowledge the following:

The recipe for Gazpacho appears in the *AMERICAN DIABETES ASSOCIATION/ AMERICAN DIETETIC ASSOCIATION FAMILY COOKBOOK, VOLUME I*, Copyright © 1980 by American Diabetes Association, Inc., The American Dietetic Association. Used by permission of the publisher, Prentice Hall, Inc., Englewood Cliffs, New Jersey.

The recipes for Fluffy High-Fiber, Low-Fat Pancakes; Herbed Pork Kabobs; and Pepper Steak appear in the *AMERICAN DIABETES ASSOCIATION/AMERICAN DIETETIC ASSOCIATION FAMILY COOKBOOK, VOLUME II*, Copyright © 1984 by American Diabetes Association, Inc., The American Dietetic Association. Used by permission of the publisher, Prentice Hall, Inc., Englewood Cliffs, New Jersey.

The recipe for Noodle Pudding appears in the *AMERICAN DIABETES ASSOCIA- TION HOLIDAY COOKBOOK* by Betty Wedman, M.S., R.D., Copyright © 1986 American Diabetes Association, Inc.

The recipes for Chocolate Angel Food Cake and Spicy/Hot Black-Eyed Peas were published in *SOUTHERN LIVING*® magazine. Used by permission of *SOUTHERN LIVING*® magazine.

All other recipes were published in *Diabetes Forecast*, ADA's monthly magazine on living better with diabetes, or were developed by the creators of *Month of Meals 2*.

For information on ordering any of the cookbooks mentioned above or joining the American Diabetes Association, call the ADA National Center at 1-800-ADA-DISC or contact your state ADA affiliate, listed in the white pages of the phone book.

People with diabetes can eat a wide variety of foods — including packaged foods, such as frozen entrees — as long as their overall diet is well-balanced. Therefore, as a convenient aid to readers who want fast yet healthy meal choices, *Month of Meals 2* includes a number of brand- or product names. The use of selected brand names does not imply that they are the only brands in a product category suitable for people with diabetes. In addition, although every attempt possible was made to ensure that these packaged foods meet calorie restrictions of individual menus, the American Diabetes Association does not endorse these products or guarantee that they are appropriate for all people with diabetes. Consumers are encouraged to read food labels carefully and to consult with a health-care professional to decide whether a food is appropriate for their meal plans.

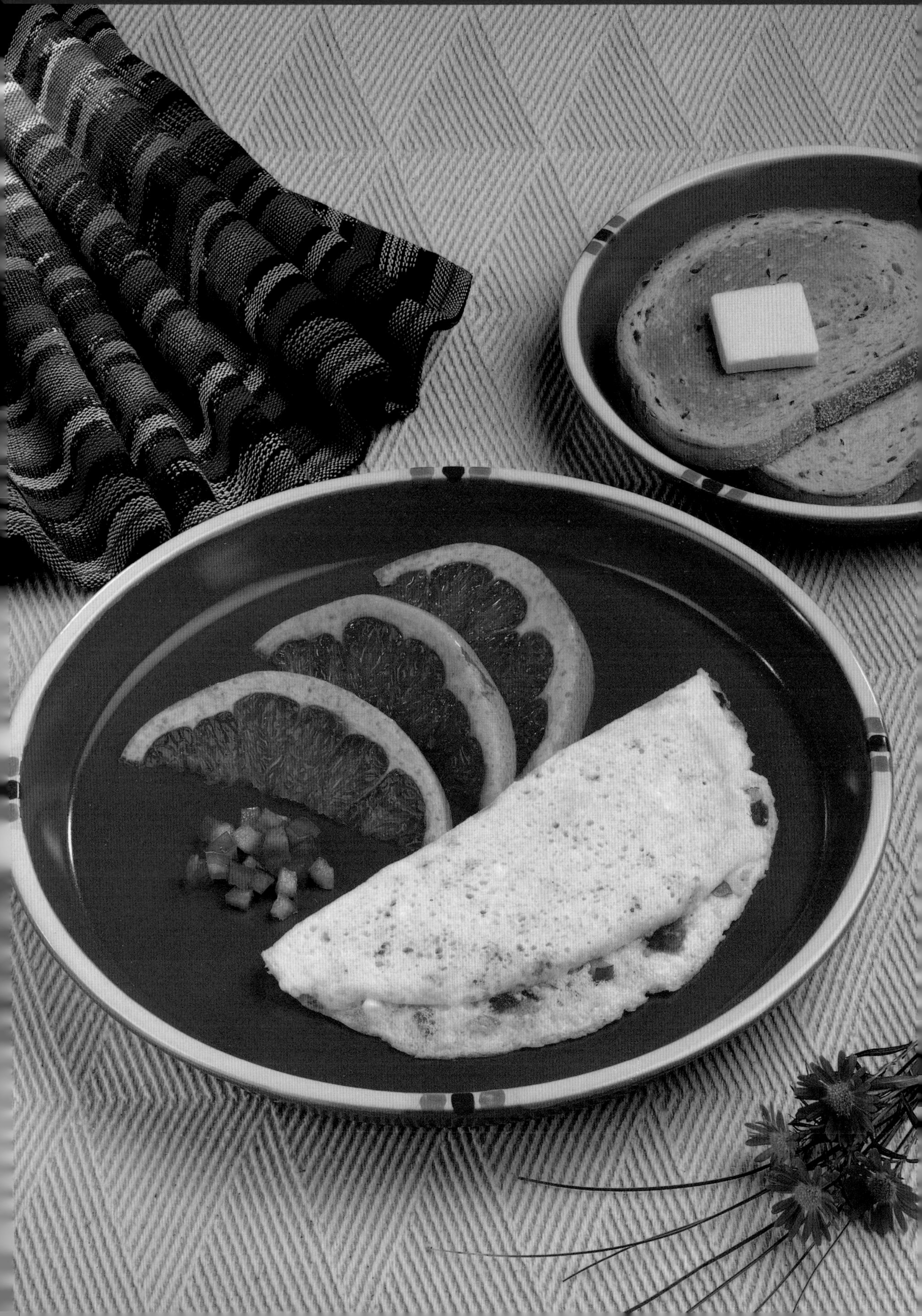

INTRODUCTION

Welcome to *Month of Meals 2*. This book is designed to help you choose healthy foods and prepare quick and easy meals. There are complete menus for breakfast, lunch, dinner, and snacks. You'll find many menus that can be prepared in less than 30 minutes, plus menus planned around ethnic cuisine and convenience foods. The book is set up in a way that will allow you to mix and match meals for a month.

Each day's menu — breakfast, lunch, dinner, and a snack — provides approximately 1500 calories. This figure can be adjusted up or down to meet your specific calorie requirements. A day's menus will provide about 45 to 50 percent of the calories from carbohydrate, 20 percent from protein, and about 30 percent from fat.

Good nutrition means eating a variety of foods from all the six food groups. Daily menus in *Month of Meals 2* provide well-balanced — and tasty — meals. The book also follows other guidelines that help you make healthy food choices:

- **Eat less fat.** *Month of Meals 2* uses low-fat meals and recommends using such products as reduced- or low-calorie salad dressings. The menus also average less than 300 milligrams of cholesterol per day.

- **Eat more high-fiber foods.** Many meals incorporate high-fiber foods: fruits; vegetables; legumes, such as beans, peas, and lentils; and whole-grain breads, cereals, and crackers.

- **Eat less sugar.** The book uses recipes that are low in sugar. No-sugar or low-sugar fruit spreads (jams or jellies) are recommended. Simple desserts containing limited amounts of sugar are included.

Instead of sugar, you can also use sweeteners that are non-caloric, such as aspartame (Equal® or NutraSweet®), acesulfame-K (Sweet One® or Sunette®), and saccharin (Sweet 'n Low®, Sugar Twin®, or Sweet 10®).

- **Use less salt**. The menus in the book will help you keep your total day's intake of sodium between 2000 and 3000 milligrams. Be sure to taste the food before you salt it! You may not need any salt at all. We've tried to use a variety of spices and herbs to enhance the natural flavors in the food.

THE SIX FOOD GROUPS

The menus in *Month of Meals 2* have been developed using a meal planning system that divides foods into six groups: Starch/Bread, Meat and Meat substitutes, Vegetables, Fruit, Milk, and Fat. Foods are placed into one group or another based on their nutrient make-up of carbohydrate, protein, fat, and calories.

Starch/Bread. This group includes cereal, pasta, rice, breads, starchy vegetables, crackers, and many snack-type foods.

Meat and Substitutes. This group includes beef, pork, lamb, veal, poultry, fish, seafood, eggs, cheese, and peanut butter. The list divides these foods into lean, medium-fat, and high-fat choices.

Vegetables. The vegetable list is made up of nonstarchy vegetables that are either cooked or raw.

Fruit. This list includes all varieties of fruit — fresh, frozen, canned, and dried, as well as fruit juices.

Milk. This list includes milk, plus yogurt and buttermilk.

Fat. Here you will find obvious fats like margarine, butter, cooking oils, mayonnaise, and salad dressings, plus other high-fat foods like avocados, olives, nuts and seeds, bacon, sour cream, and cream cheese.

For a complete listing of foods and portion sizes in the six food groups, see *Exchange Lists for Meal Planning*, available from the American Diabetes Association or The American Dietetic Association.

Food Group	Calories Per Serving
Starch/Bread	80
Meat and Substitutes	
Lean	55
Medium-Fat	75
High-Fat	100
Vegetables	25
Fruit	60
Milk	
Skim	90
Low-Fat	120
Whole	150
Fat	45

A D D I N G   V A R I E T Y   T O   M E A L   P L A N N I N G

The menus in *Month of Meals 2* include plenty of variety, more mixed dishes, and many ethnic foods. You may, however, still want to substitute some of your favorite recipes for recipes listed on the menus. Here are guidelines to help you make substitutions.

Casseroles. Want to use your own homemade casserole or spaghetti dish instead of the ones listed in this book? That's easy. Substitute one cup of your favorite casserole recipe for the casserole listed in the *Month of Meals 2* menu. One cup of many homemade casseroles averages between 300 to 350 calories (2 Starch/Bread, 2 Medium-Fat Meat, and 0 to 1 Fat servings).

Substitute any of these food choices:

- 1 cup beef and vegetable stew (with potato)
- 1 cup chili with beans
- 1 cup macaroni and cheese
- 2 cups chicken chow mein
- 1/4 of a 10-inch diameter (about 15 oz.) thin crust, cheese pizza
- 1 cup spaghetti and meat balls
- 1 cup tuna noodle casserole
- 1 cup goulash

Soups. You may substitute other soups for those listed in the menus if you stay within your calorie requirements. One cup of a broth-type/vegetable soup averages 75 to 80 calories (1 Starch/Bread serving). One cup of a canned cream soup made with water averages 100 to 110 calories (1 Starch/Bread and 1 Fat serving). One cup of a canned bean soup made with water averages 175 calories (1 Starch/Bread, 1 Lean-Meat, and 1 Vegetable serving).

Substitute any of these soup choices:

Broth-type soups/vegetable soups
- 1 cup vegetarian vegetable or vegetable with beef
- 1 cup chicken rice
- 1 cup chicken or beef noodle
- 1 cup gumbo

Cream soups
- 1 cup cream of asparagus, chicken, potato, or tomato
- 1 cup New England clam chowder

Bean soups
- 1 cup bean with bacon
- 1 cup black bean
- 1 cup split pea

Vegetarian Meals. Vegetables are an excellent source of vitamins, minerals, protein, and fiber. What's more, vegetarian meals are usually low in fat, especially saturated fats and cholesterol.

Lunch menus 8, 23, 25, and 26 and dinner menus 3, 15, and 22 are examples of vegetarian meals.

Desserts. Moderate amounts of some foods can be used, even if they do contain some sugar. In general, sugar in recipes is limited to approximately 1 teaspoon per serving. If a serving contains 1 teaspoon to 1 tablespoon of sugar per serving, it is recommended for occasional use only. If a dessert has more than 1 tablespoon of sugar per serving, it is not recommended.

Working sweet desserts into your meal plan means making the right substitutions. Here's a handy list to help.

- 2 small cookies or 1 medium-size cookie averages 80 to 120 calories (1 Starch/Bread and 1 Fat serving)

- 1 small serving of cake without frosting averages 200 to 250 calories per serving (2 Starch/Bread and 1 to 2 Fat servings)

- 1/12 angel food cake is 150 calories (2 Starch/Bread servings)

- 1/12 9-inch sponge cake is 150 to 200 calories (1 1/2 Starch/Bread and 1 Fat serving)

- 1/12 9-inch chocolate, white, or yellow cake is 250 calories (2 Starch/Bread and 2 Fat servings)

- 1/2 cup of ice cream averages 130 to 150 calories (1 Starch/Bread and 2 Fat servings)

- 1/2 cup ice milk averages 100 to 110 calories (1 Starch/Bread and 1 Fat serving)

- 1/4 cup sherbet or Italian fruit ice averages 70 to 80 calories (1 Starch/Bread serving)

- 1/3 cup frozen yogurt averages 80 calories (1 Starch/Bread serving)

Packaged Convenience Foods. Today, we have many more frozen entrees or frozen convenience meals to choose from. They may be "light," "lite," lower calorie, or calorie-controlled. You may choose to use these for a quick dinner or lunch.

Look for meals that meet these guidelines:

- 300 calories or less
- 15 grams of fat or less per entree or meal
- 100 milligrams of cholesterol or less
- 800 milligrams of sodium or less.

Add a serving of fresh fruit or a glass of skim milk, a tossed green salad with reduced-calorie dressing, and a slice of whole-wheat bread or roll and you still have a meal under 550 calories.

These guidelines are best used when selecting a frozen dinner that includes an entree and side dishes. If you choose just an entree, you will need to add more food to round out the meal.

See lunch menus 2, 5, and 12 and dinner menus 6 and 18 for ideas on how to use convenience foods. Convenience foods are marked with the symbol 🔲

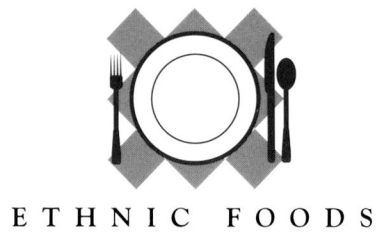

ETHNIC FOODS

Add variety, interest, and spice to your meal plan with ethnic foods. But take care. Sometimes ethnic foods can be high in calories, fat, and salt. That's why some recipes may need to be modified. Here are guidelines to follow:

Mexican Foods. Many Mexican dishes resemble stews or casseroles. Instead of separate servings of meat, starch, and vegetables, meat is usually added to potatoes, chili peppers, tomatoes, and other foods to make one dish. So, look carefully at the total calories and use the casserole guidelines on page 5.

Salsa — red or green chili sauce — is a favorite. It is made of finely diced tomatoes, chili peppers, and onions. Salsa adds spice to a meal — with very few calories.

Beans, tortillas, Spanish rice, noodles, and potatoes are good sources of carbohydrates and are excellent side dishes for any meal plan. Beans are also high in fiber. Use them, but don't fry or refry them — as is traditional — in lard. Instead, cook beans by boiling them. Watch portion sizes of high-fat cheeses, such as Cheddar and Monterey Jack. Choose cheeses made from skim milk or with 5 grams or less of fat per ounce, such as part-skim mozzarella, Farmer's, or string cheeses.

See lunch menus 1 and 25 and dinner menus 4, 5, 22, and 23 Mexican-style foods.

Italian Foods. Think of pasta, tomatoes, veal, cheese, olive oil, and fresh herbs and you think Italian. By using pasta, tomatoes and artichokes, low-fat cheeses, and small portions of meat, Italian cooking can meet your nutritional goals.

Traditional spices like basil, rosemary, oregano, and garlic will add zest to the meal. Using olive oil is another health advantage, but be sure to watch portions. Remember, 1 tablespoon of oil contains 120 calories. As for desserts, keep them simple with fresh fruits, small servings of cheese, and fruit ices.

See lunch menus 8, 20, and 24, and dinner menus 3, 21, and 28 for Italian flair.

Jewish Foods. When you think of Jewish foods, you often think of dark rye breads, borscht, and herring. But eggplant, humus, kasha, and couscous are other favorites.

Traditionally, large portions of breads, noodles, cooked beans and peas, and pastries are eaten. So, when choosing Jewish foods, watch portion sizes. Also watch the amount of high-fat meats — corned beef, pastrami, well-marbled cuts of meats, or chicken fat (schmaltz) — you eat. Many of these high-fat meats are highly salted as well. Instead, choose lean cuts of meats, such as flank steak, top round, or extra lean ground beef. Use non-fat yogurt instead of sour cream and blended low-fat cottage cheese or light cream cheese instead of regular cream cheese.

See lunch menu 6 and dinner menu 9 for Jewish meals.

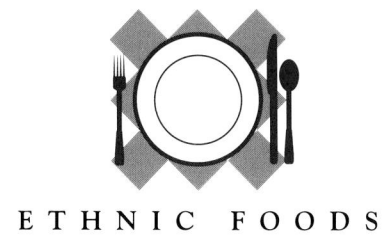

ETHNIC FOODS

Oriental Foods. Vegetables and fruits are used abundantly in Oriental cooking. Vegetables are rarely eaten raw. Instead, they are stir-fried, steamed, or added to soups. A wide variety of meats, often pork, poultry, and seafood, are used in small portions in Oriental dishes. Rice is a staple in the diet and accompanies almost every meal. Soybeans, like other legumes, are used dried or as sprouts. They are also made into tofu, which can be stir-fried, braised, or fermented into sauces for seasoning. Peanut oil and corn oil are commonly used for stir-frying.

Oriental foods are often marinated or pre-seasoned with condiments, such as soy sauce, oyster sauce, or bean paste — all high in sodium. Preserved foods, such as salted fish and eggs, pickled vegetables, and sausages, are also extremely high in sodium. Low-sodium seasoning alternatives include ginger, garlic, and scallions.

Dinner menus 8, 19, and 25 provide tasty foods with Oriental flavor.

Month of Meals 2 allows you to choose the calorie level that best meets your nutritional needs. First, however, you need to know about how many daily calories you require. The best way to do this is to meet with a dietitian who can design a meal plan with the right number of calories for you.

Basic Meal Plan
1500 Calories A Day
Each breakfast, lunch, and dinner in Month of Meals 2 has about the same number of calories, so you can mix and match them to suit your own tastes. One days' breakfast, lunch, and dinner total is about 1350 calories. By adding two 60-calorie snacks OR one 125-calorie snack, your daily total will be 1500 calories — the Basic Meal Plan. Choose any menus you like. All the portions on the menus are for one person, so you can have everything listed.

If you need more or less calories than the basic 1500 menus provide, no problem. Adjusting meals to meet your requirements is as easy as following the instructions on the next few pages.

Basic Meal Plan Plus
If you are following a meal plan that allows you 1800 calories a day, use the chart below to adjust the basic meal plan.

First, choose any menu in Month of Meals 2 that you want. Then, move down the 1800-calorie column and follow the directions: Breakfast is the same as the Basic Meal Plan — plus one 125-calorie morning snack. Lunch is the same as the Basic Meal Plan — plus one 125-calorie afternoon snack. Dinner is the same as the Basic Meal Plan — plus one 170-calorie evening snack.

The chart shows you how to reach an 1800- and a 2100-calorie meal plan.

	BASIC MEAL PLAN 1500 CALORIES	1800 CALORIES	2100 CALORIES
Breakfast	Total calories: 350	Same as Basic Meal Plan Total calories: 350	Add one meat OR one Starch/Bread to the Basic Meal Plan Total calories: 425
Morning Snack		Add one 125-calorie snack Total calories: 125	Add one 60-calorie snack Total calories: 60
Lunch	Total calories: 450	Same as Basic Meal Plan Total calories: 450	Add one Starch/Bread AND one Fat to the Basic Meal Plan Total calories: 575
Afternoon Snack		Add one 125-calorie snack Total calories: 125	Add one 125-calorie snack Total calories: 125
Dinner	Total calories: 550	Same as Basic Meal Plan Total calories: 550	Add one Starch/Bread AND one Milk to the Basic Meal Plan Total calories: 720
Evening Snack	Two 60-calorie snacks OR one 125-calorie snack Total calories: 125	Add one 170-calorie snack Total calories: 170	Add one 170-calorie snack Total calories: 170

Basic Meal Plan Minus*

If you are following a meal plan that allows you 1200 calories a day, use the chart below to adjust the basic meal plan.

First, choose any menu in *Month of Meals 2* that you want. Then, move down the 1200-calorie column and follow the directions: Eliminate one starch or one milk for breakfast from the Basic Meal Plan. Eliminate one fruit at lunch from the Basic Meal Plan. Eliminate one fat at dinner from the Basic Meal Plan. No snacks.

This chart shows you how to reach a 1200- and a 1350-calorie meal plan.

*To meet your body's most basic nutrient needs, you need to eat at least 1200 calories a day.

	1200 CALORIES	1350 CALORIES	BASIC MEAL PLAN 1500 CALORIES
Breakfast	Eliminate one Starch/Bread or one Milk from Basic Meal Plan Total calories: **270**	Same as Basic Meal Plan Total calories: **350**	Total calories: **350**
Morning Snack			
Lunch	Eliminate one Fruit from Basic Meal Plan Total calories: **390**	Same as Basic Meal Plan Total calories: **450**	Total calories: **450**
Afternoon Snack			
Dinner	Eliminate one Fat from Basic Meal Plan Total calories: **505**	Same as Basic Meal Plan Total calories: **550**	Total calories: **550**
Evening Snack			Two 60-calorie snacks OR one 125-calorie snack Total calories: **125**

Sample Meal Plan #1

Here's how to adjust the Basic Meal Plan (1500 calories) for about a 1200-calorie diet.

Meal	Calories
Breakfast	350
Plus or minus	
−1 **Starch/Bread** serving(s)	−80
# (type of serving)	Subtotal 270
Lunch	450
Plus or minus	
−1 **Fruit** serving(s)	−60
# (type of serving)	Subtotal 390
Dinner	550
Plus or minus	
−1 **Fat** serving(s)	−45
# (type of serving)	Subtotal 505
	TOTAL DAILY CALORIES 1165

Sample Meal Plan #2

Here's how to adjust the Basic Meal Plan (1500 calories) for about a 2200-calorie diet.

Meal	Calories
Breakfast	350
Plus or minus	
+1 **Starch/Bread** serving(s)	+80
# (type of serving)	Subtotal 430
Lunch	450
Plus or minus	
+1 **Fruit** serving(s)	+60
# (type of serving)	
+1 **Fat** serving(s)	+45
# (type of serving)	Subtotal 555
Dinner	550
Plus or minus	
+1 **Starch/Bread** serving(s)	+80
# (type of serving)	
+1 **Med-Fat Meat** servings(s)	+75
# (type of serving)	
+1 **Fat** serving(s)	+45
# (type of serving)	Subtotal 750
Snacks (Morning, Afternoon , and/or Evening)	420
+1 **Fruit** serving(s)	+60
# (type of serving)	Subtotal 480
	TOTAL DAILY CALORIES 2215

Your Meal Plan

Meal	Calories

Breakfast _____

Plus or minus

___ _____ serving(s) _____

\#   (type of serving)   Subtotal _____

Morning Snack

___ _____ serving(s) _____

\#   (type of serving)   Subtotal _____

Lunch _____

Plus or minus

___ _____ serving(s) _____

\#   (type of serving)

___ _____ serving(s) _____

\#   (type of serving)   Subtotal _____

Afternoon Snack

___ _____ serving(s) _____

\#   (type of serving)   Subtotal _____

Dinner _____

Plus or minus

___ _____ serving(s) _____

\#   (type of serving)

___ _____ serving(s) _____

\#   (type of serving)

___ _____ serving(s) _____

\#   (type of serving)   Subtotal _____

Evening Snack

___ _____ serving(s) _____

\#   (type of serving)   Subtotal _____

TOTAL DAILY CALORIES _____

HOW TO USE THIS BOOK

Just like in the original *Month of Meals*, the pages in this book are divided into thirds so that each menu (breakfast, lunch, or dinner) appears on a separate segment. You can either follow each day's meal plan in sequence or flip back and forth between the various menus for added variety.

For example, on one day you may have Breakfast 3, Lunch 2, Dinner 26, and Snack 12 for a total of 1500 calories.

Most of the breakfasts and lunches can be prepared quickly. Many of the dinners, too, are quick and easy. If you are in a hurry, the following dinners are quick choices: 1, 2, 5, 6, 7, 11, 16, 18, 26, and 27. Quick-choice meals are marked with the symbol ⊙.

Many recipes in this book yield more than the one serving called for in the menus. The total number of servings (yield) and the single serving size are listed at the top of each recipe.

To handle leftovers:

- Avoid leftovers altogether by preparing the recipes in *Month of Meals 2* for the whole family. Then, everyone can get the benefits of eating right, and you won't feel isolated or deprived by having to eat "special meals."

- If you're preparing meals for just yourself or for two people, divide leftovers into individual portions and freeze for later use. Be sure to use materials designed for freezer use — plastic storage bags — and mark the packages clearly with the date and contents.

- Store breads or other dry leftovers in air-tight containers or plastic storage bags.

Recipes in this book use these standard abbreviations:

> Tbsp. = Tablespoon
> tsp. = teaspoon
> oz. = ounce
> lb. = pound

Tips for Healthy Eating
You may:

- use commercial (canned or dry) or home-made soups with these menus.

- use no-sugar or low-sugar fruit spreads (jams or jellies). Limit yourself to 1 to 2 teaspoons (less than 20 calories) per serving.

- use 1 teaspoon of regular margarine or 1 Tablespoon of diet margarine interchangeably.

- use 1 Tablespoon of regular salad dressing or 2 Tablespoons of reduced-calorie salad dressing interchangeably. (These menus use reduced-calorie salad dressing.)

- have free raw vegetables on some menus, which can include salad greens and moderate servings of carrot or celery sticks, tomatoes, cucumbers, green pepper slices, radishes, and the like.

- use butter-flavored granules, such as Butter Buds® or Molly McButter®, to season vegetables, potatoes, rice, or noodles.

- add your choice of calorie-free beverages, such as coffee, hot or iced tea, mineral water, diet sodas.

- use skim or 1% milk in all menus and recipes.

- measure meat portions after cooking. Four ounces of uncooked meat shrinks to about three ounces after cooking.

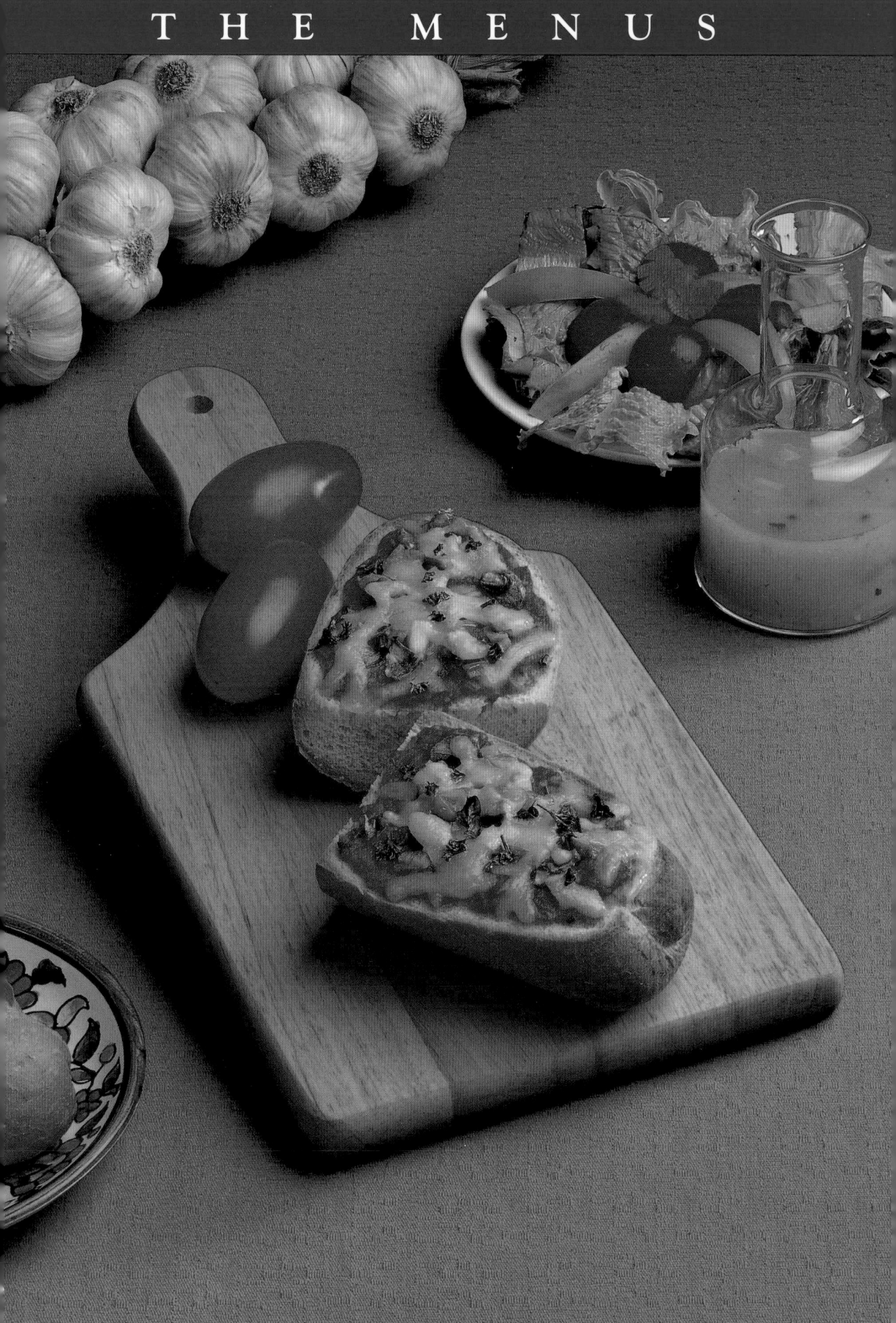

Each **breakfast** in this section has about **350 calories** and includes:

2	Starch/Bread	servings
1	Fruit	serving
1	Skim Milk	serving
1	Fat	serving

In some menus, one Meat serving has been used in place of either the Skim Milk serving or one of the Starch/Bread servings.

Each **lunch** in this section has about **450 calories** and includes:

2	Starch/Bread	servings
2	Meat	servings
0-1	Vegetable	serving
1	Fruit	serving
1	Fat	serving

In some menus, one Milk serving has been used in place of either one of the Meat or Starch/Bread servings.

Each **dinner** in this section has about **550 calories** and includes:

2	Starch/Bread	servings
3	Meat	servings
1-2	Vegetable	servings
1	Fruit	serving
2	Fat	servings

In some menus, one Milk serving has been used in place of either one of the Meat or Starch/Bread servings.

Breakfast #7
SPANISH OMELETTE (Continued)
Method

1. In nonstick skillet, saute green pepper, onion, and garlic in water. Add chopped chili, tomato, and pimento and boil off remaining liquid.
2. Combine egg whites and saffron and beat into soft peaks. Fold cottage cheese into egg whites, followed by the contents of the skillet.
3. Return to skillet and fry until eggs are set, turning to avoid scorching. Pour off any water rendered during cooking and serve.

Breakfast #23
BROCCOLI QUICHE (Continued)
Method

1. Cook broccoli according to package directions; drain.
2. Place broccoli in 9-inch pie plate sprayed with nonstick vegetable cooking spray; sprinkle with green pepper, onion, and cheese. Set aside.
3. Combine remaining ingredients in container of electric blender; blend 15 seconds or until smooth.
4. Pour over broccoli mixture; bake at 375 degrees for 25 to 30 minutes or until set. Let stand 5 minutes before serving.

Lunch #25
STUFFED PEPPERS MEXICALI
(Continued)

2. Add the tofu and saute until brown. Add the tomatoes, corn, and seasonings. Cook covered for 5 minutes over low heat.
3. Slightly mash the beans. Add to the tofu-vegetable mixture. Stir.
4. Cut the peppers in half lengthwise and remove the seeds. Leave the stems on to help the pepper halves retain their shape during baking.
5. Fill each half pepper full of the tofu-vegetable mixture. Grate cheese on top of peppers. Prepare a pan with nonstick vegetable cooking spray. Put 1/2-inch of tomato juice or water on the bottom of the pan and place pepper halves in the liquid.
6. Cover tightly, and bake at 375 degrees for 30 to 40 minutes. Garnish with hot sauce, if desired.

Dinner #1
SPINACH MANICOTTI (Continued)
Method

1. Cook manicotti shells according to package directions, omitting salt; drain and set aside.
2. Combine next 8 ingredients; cover and cook sauce over low heat for 1 hour.
3. Cook spinach according to package directions, omitting salt. Drain; place on paper towels and squeeze until barely moist. Combine spinach, cottage cheese, Parmesan cheese, and nutmeg. Stuff manicotti shells with spinach mixture and arrange in a 13- by 9- by 2-inch baking dish coated with cooking spray.
4. Pour tomato sauce over manicotti. Bake at 350 degrees for 45 minutes. Garnish with parsley.

Dinner #4
CHICKEN FAJITA (Continued)
Saute, stirring occasionally until onion is slightly brown, but still crisp and tender.

4. Grill chicken in another nonstick skillet with only a small amount of oil, until no longer pink. Serve with onions and green peppers on tortilla.

Breakfast #26
FLUFFY HIGH-FIBER, LOW-FAT PAN-CAKES (Continued)
Method

1. Combine buttermilk, oats, and bran in large mixing bowl. Let stand 5 minutes. Add egg and beat until blended.
2. Mix whole-wheat flour, sugar, salt, and baking soda until blended.
3. Add to bran mixture and blend until all flour is moistened.

4. Pour about 1/4-cup batter on lightly greased, preheated 375-degree frying pan. Cook about 3 minutes or until bubbles form and the edge of pancake is dry. Turn and cook 2 minutes longer. This is a "fat" pancake.
5. Top with 1/2 cup strawberry topping. To make strawberry topping, place 1 cup strawberries and 1 tsp. apple juice concentrate in blender. Blend until smooth.

Dinner #8
TURKEY POLYNESIAN (Continued)
Method

1. In small bowl, combine cornstarch, water, soy sauce, and salt. Mix well. Coat turkey cubes with cornstarch mixture.
2. In nonstick skillet over medium heat, saute onions in 1 tsp. oil.
3. Add celery, water chestnuts, and snow peas. Cook for 2 minutes. Remove vegetables from skillet.
4. To skillet, add 1 tsp. oil and turkey. Saute until brown. Add sauteed vegetables, pineapple, and juice. Simmer for 10 minutes. Remove from heat. Add oranges. Serve over hot rice.

Dinner #10
CHICKEN WITH SUN-DRIED TOMA-TOES (Continued)

Add broth, wine (much of the alcohol will evaporate, leaving the flavor), marjoram, and sun-dried tomatoes.
4. Bring to a boil over moderate heat and cook, uncovered, 5 minutes, stirring occasionally.
5. Return the chicken to the skillet. Simmer, gently spooning the sauce over the chicken, until heated through. Simmer until the sauce is reduced by half.

Dinner #12
HERBED PORK KABOBS (Continued)
4. Cut pork into 1 1/2-inch cubes and thread on 4 skewers.
5. Place on wire rack over shallow baking dish. Broil 4 inches from heat. Turn frequently; baste occasionally with herb-butter mix until brown on all sides. Serve with lemon wedges.

Dinner #17
CHICKEN OKRA GUMBO (Continued)
3. In a 6-quart kettle, make a roux by adding 1/4 cup flour to the reserved cooking fat, stirring constantly over low heat until it is light brown, but not burnt.
4. Add water, salt, pepper, and vegetables. Stir a few minutes. Add fried chicken. Cook for about 1 hour or until chicken is tender.

Dinner #19
PORK CHOP ORIENTAL (Continued)
4. Cover and refrigerate 1 1/2 hours, turning once after about 45 minutes.
5. Heat the broiler. Shake the garlic from the chops, and sprinkle both sides with pepper. Place in the preheated broiler and broil for 5 minutes on each side, or until browned outside and still moist inside.

Dinner #20
CHICKEN CASSEROLE (Continued)
3. In medium mixing bowl, combine chicken, broccoli, and onion. Stir in sauce and mix well to coat all ingredients.
4. Pour into 1 quart casserole. Top with toasted oats. Bake for 30 minutes at 350 degrees.

Dinner #21
CHOCOLATE ANGELFOOD CAKE (Continued)
Yield: 32 1/2-inch servings /Serving Size: 1 serving

Ingredients
1 14.5-oz. angel food cake mix
1/4 cup unsweetened cocoa, sifted
1/4 tsp. chocolate flavoring
1 Tbsp. powdered sugar, sifted
Method
1. Combine flour packet from cake mix with cocoa. Prepare cake according to package directions; fold chocolate flavoring into batter. Bake according to package directions. Sprinkle cooled cake with powdered sugar.

Dinner #22
VEGETABLE CHILI (Continued)
Method
1. In a large nonstick skillet, heat oil until hot. Add onion and garlic. Saute until lightly browned, about 3 minutes.
2. Add tomatoes with liquid, green peppers, zucchini, chili powder, oregano, cumin, and black pepper.
3. Simmer, covered, until vegetables are tender, about 15 minutes.
4. Combine flour with water. Add to chili along with kidney beans. Cook and stir until thickened, about 5 minutes.

DINNER

DINNER

Dinner #23
TAMALE PIE (Continued)

4. Prepare corn bread mix according to package instructions. Divide 1 cup of corn bread batter into four equal portions. Spoon batter portions approximately 2 inches apart over the warm meat mixture.
5. Bake in preheated oven at 375 degrees for 30 to 40 minutes or until corn bread is done. Sprinkle top with paprika, and serve.

Dinner #25
KUNG PAO CHICKEN (Continued)
Method

1. Season chicken with rice wine, egg white, cornstarch, and 1 Tbsp. vegetable oil.
2. Spray wok with nonstick vegetable cooking spray. Stir-fry chicken until done.
3. Remove chicken and clean wok. Spray again with nonstick vegetable cooking spray. Add remaining 1 Tbsp. vegetable oil. Heat oil and saute garlic, green onion, chili peppers, ginger, salt, sugar, and hot sauce. Add wine and chicken. Stir and serve over rice.

Dinner #27
PEPPER STEAK (Continued)

3. Add remaining oil to skillet, heat, add steak and stir-fry 2 minutes.
4. Mix cornstarch with water, add to steak. Cook, stirring constantly until thickened. Add vegetables, mix thoroughly. Serve over rice.

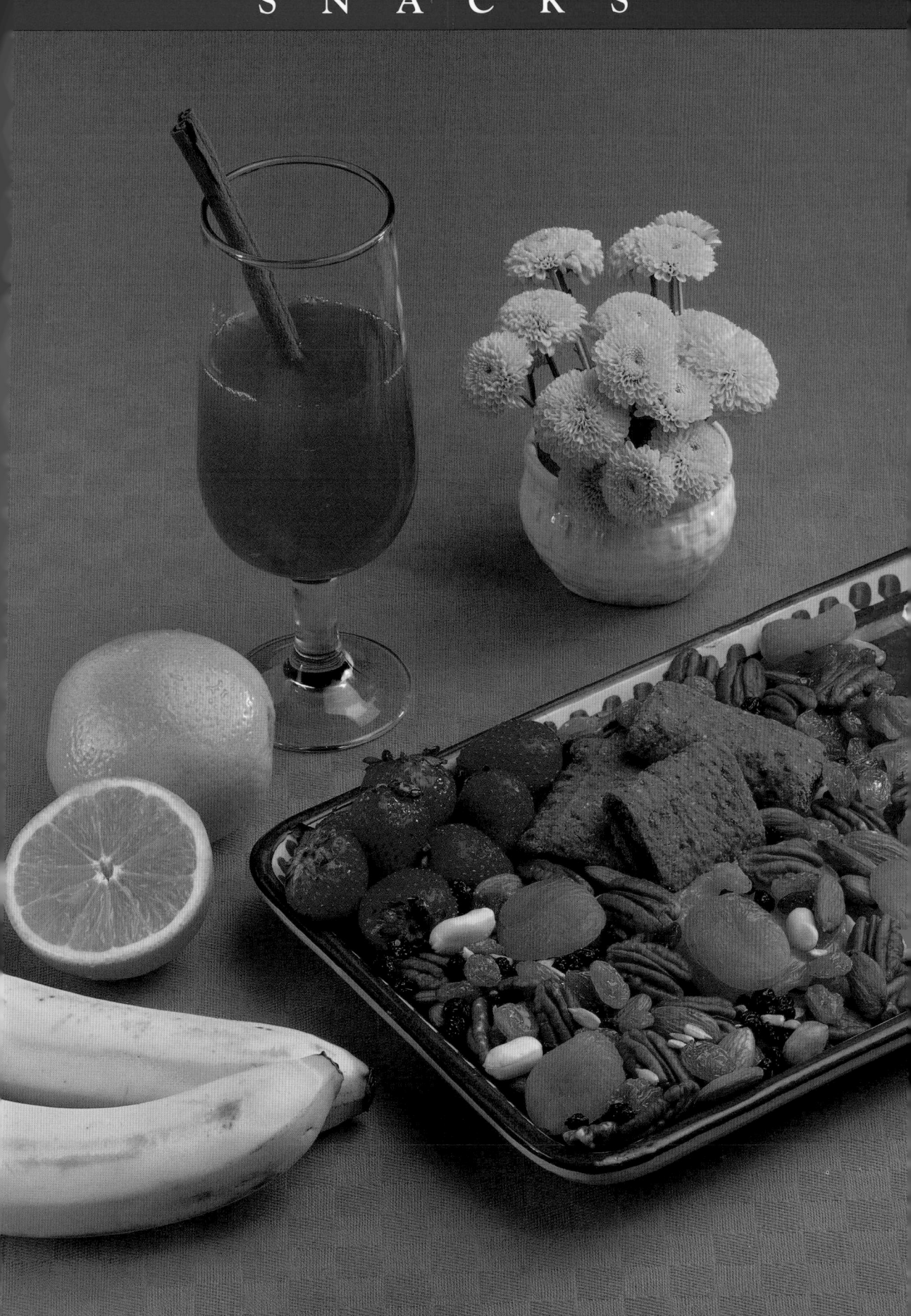

The snacks in this section are divided into three groups.

Each **60-calorie** snack equals

1 Fruit serving

Each **125-calorie** snack equals

1 Starch/Bread serving AND
1 Fat serving

Each **170-calorie** snack equals

1 Starch/Bread serving
1 Skim Milk serving OR
1 Meat serving

S N A C K S

60 calories

1
4 dried apple rings

2
3 medium prunes

3
1/2 cup strawberries
4 animal crackers

4
1 1/4 cup watermelon
cubes

5
1/3 medium cantaloupe

6
1/2 cup unsweetened
applesauce

7
1 fruit roll-up

8
1 1/2 cups V-8® juice

9
1 Dole® Fruit and Juice®
bar

10
5 oz. Sundance®
fruit Sparkler

11
1 orange, sliced,
topped with
1 tsp. sugar substitute and
1 Tbsp. lemon juice and
2 Tbsp. apple juice

12
1/2 cup apple cider

13
1/2 small banana, frozen
and sliced

14
1 cup cantaloupe cubes
sprinkled with nutmeg

15
1 fig bar cookie

16
2 plums

17
1 cup melon balls

18
2 gelatin pops

19
1 package (1/2 oz.)
Weight Watchers® Apple
Snack

20
1 Flavor Tree® Fruit Roll

21
1 bar Jello-O® Citrus
Snowburst

22
1 serving Campbell's®
Cup® of instant soup

23
1 Welch's® Fruit Juice Bar

125 calories

1
1/2 slice angel food cake topped with 1/2 cup strawberries and 1 Tbsp. whipped topping

2
1 oz. pretzels

3
1 toaster waffle 2 tsp. low-sugar fruit spread

4
3 Nabisco Lorna Doone® cookies

5
3/4 cup CornNuts®

6
1/3 cup Pepperidge Farm® Goldfish crackers

7
22 Nabisco Teddy Grahams®

8
1/2 cup Edy's Grand Light® dairy dessert

9
10 Nabisco Wheat Thins®

10
1/2 cup frozen yogurt

11
1 slice banana bread (1/16 loaf)

12
4 cups Pop Secret® Light Microwave Popcorn

13
1/2 cup vanilla ice milk 1/4 cup blueberries

14
1 cup tomato soup 4 saltine crackers

15
2 oz. boiled shrimp with 1 Tbsp. cocktail sauce 5 saltine crackers

16
3 slices cocktail rye bread, spread with 1 1/2 Tbsp. light cream cheese and topped with cucumber slice

17
1 slice French bread, broiled with 1 tsp. diet margarine, 1 Tbsp. Parmesan cheese, and basil

18
1/4 cup trail mix: raisins, nuts, dried fruit

19
10 animal crackers

20
1 Archway® Apple Filled Oatmeal Cookie

21
2 R. W. Frookie® Apple Cinnamon or Oat Bran cookies

22
6 ginger snaps

23
1 Kellogg's® Rice Krispies® Bar

24
2/3 cup Ralston® Chex® Snack Mix

170 calories

1
1 oz. Kraft Cheez Whiz®
5 slices melba toast

2
1 oz. Laughing Cow®
cheese spread
6 saltine crackers

3
1 envelope sugar-free
Carnation Instant
Breakfast®
1 cup skim milk

4
1 cup nonfat fruit-flavored
yogurt, sweetened with
sugar substitute
3 Tbsp. Post® Grape-Nuts®
cereal

5
2 rice cakes
1 Tbsp. peanut butter
2 tsp. low-sugar
fruit spread

6
2 slices French toast
2 tsp. low-sugar
fruit spread

7
1 small frozen banana with
1 Tbsp. peanut butter

8
1 pudding pop and 1 cup
skim milk

9
1/2 ham sandwich on rye
with 1 tsp. mustard

10
1/4 cup low-fat cottage
cheese
3 slices tomato
4 onion melba rounds

11
3 graham cracker squares
1 Tbsp. peanut butter

12
1/2 cup sugar-free
chocolate pudding
3 graham cracker squares

13
8 oz. sugar-free hot cocoa
3 ginger snaps

14
1 mini pizza:
1/2 English muffin
2 tsp. pizza sauce
1 oz. part-skim mozzarella
cheese

15
1/2 cup low-fat vanilla
dairy dessert
20 small pretzels

16
3/4 cup vanilla
sugar-free pudding
1/2 cup raspberries, fresh
or frozen, unsweetened
(*Layer pudding and raspberries in a parfait glass.*)

17
3/4 cup chocolate sugar-
free pudding
1/2 cup canned
unsweetened cherries or
12 fresh cherries
(*Layer pudding and cherries
in a parfait glass.*)

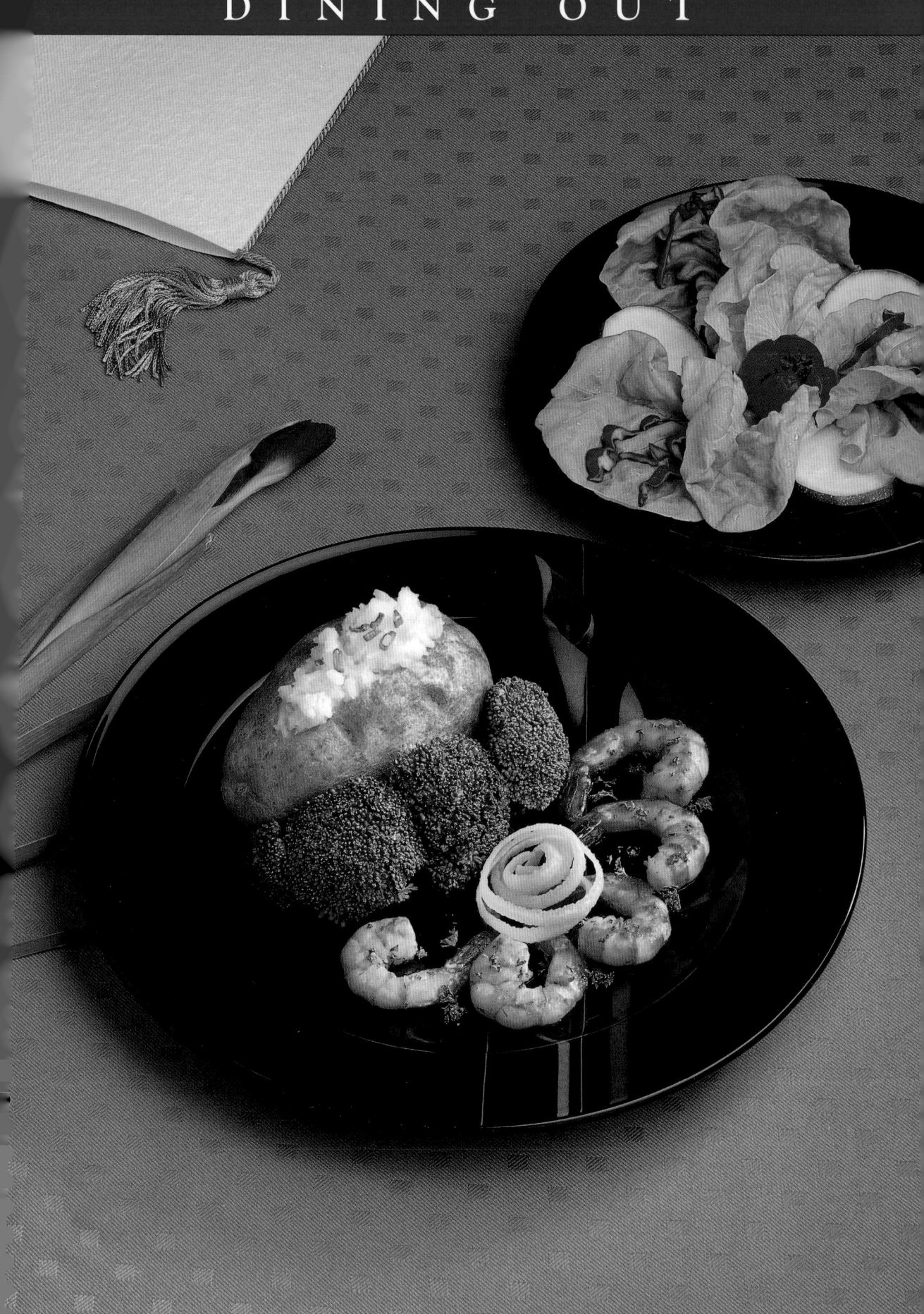

DINING OUT

Making healthy food choices when eating out begins with a decision to give up some of the high-fat menu choices and replace them with some just-as-tasty lower fat foods.

Before you even select a restaurant, make sure you are familiar with your meal plan and the number of servings from each food group that you can select. Then, call the restaurant and ask about their menu selections. Most restaurants are pleased to grant reasonable requests.

Decide ahead of time what you will order. That way you are less apt to be swayed by specials that may be too high in fat and calories or too large in portion sizes. It's helpful if your dining companions are also supportive of your desire to continue on your meal plan when eating out.

If with a group, order first. This will prevent you from being swayed by what the rest of your dining companions are ordering. At a buffet or cafeteria, select your food choices and move away from the food serving area.

Try to eat similar-sized portions to those you eat at home. If portion sizes are too large for you, try sharing portions with your dining partner. Or ask for a "doggie" bag. Ask for the bag *before* you start eating. Remove the excess food from your plate. Then sit back and enjoy. Take the extra portions home for lunch the next day.

Enjoy the company of your dining associates and the dining environment even if you must limit food choices.

DINING OUT MEXICAN STYLE

Look on the menu of many American restaurants and you're likely to see Mexican fare, from chili con carne with chips to Mexican salads. Mid-price range Mexican food chains feature nachos, tacos, enchiladas, and chili con carne, while more upscale dining establishments serve entrees such as arroz con pollo and camarones de hacha.

DINING TIPS

- Ask the waiter NOT to bring the usual basket of chips. If you should succumb to the chips, hold the melted cheese, sour cream, and guacamole. Use plain salsa instead.
- Want an appetizer? Try a salad. No grated cheese, please. Use the salsa as a reduced-calorie salad dressing. Additional appetizers to try: gazpacho, ceviche, a cup of chili con carne without the cheese, or a cup of black bean soup.
- Skip the refried beans; they are often refried in lard. Ask for black beans and a side order of Mexican rice or more tortillas instead.
- Great entrees are: chicken or beef enchiladas or burritos. Chicken or beef fajitas fit the bill, too. Try a Mexican salad topped with spicy beef or chicken.
- In general, use minimal amounts of sour cream, guacamole, cheese, and olives. Ask for them to be served on the side, if possible, or delete them entirely from your meal.

MEALS THAT PLEASE

350 CALORIES
1 bowl (1 1/2 cups) chili con carne
Tossed salad with salsa for dressing
Diet soda

375 CALORIES
2 tacos
1 packet of taco sauce
Mineral water

400 CALORIES
Chicken fajitas:
    3 oz. of chicken
    2 tortillas
    Grilled onions and peppers
Tossed salad with
1 Tablespoon reduced-calorie salad dressing

400 CALORIES
1 beef burrito
Salsa sauce
Iced tea

500 CALORIES
Taco salad:
    Shredded chicken
    Lettuce
    Onions
    Tomatoes
    Black beans
    Salsa sauce
10 taco chips
Diet soda

DINING OUT ITALIAN STYLE

Italian cuisine lends itself easily to good nutrition and healthy eating habits. All you need are a few creative strategies to lighten the calorie load.

Start by saying no to the great quantity of bread that is usually placed before you. You may ask that bread be removed from the table. If your meal plan allows, take one piece, try your best to avoid the butter, and pass the bread to the other end of the table. Don't order garlic bread. It's usually loaded with butter.

Even before you start eating, separate what you plan to eat and what you will take home. If items are not well described on the menu, ask about preparation methods.

DINING TIPS

- Salad is usually featured with pasta and/or entrees and can be a delightful "filler-upper." Always ask for dressing on the side, so you can monitor the amount used. If you are limiting calories, try lemon wedges or plain vinegar, or bring along your own individually packaged, reduced-calorie salad dressing.
- Choose the veggies on the antipasto tray and avoid the salami and olives.
- Think about sharing a pasta dish and a fish or shrimp dish with your dinner partner. Some restaurants allow you to order a luncheon-size order (half the supper portion).
- If you are ordering a pasta dish as your entree, avoid cream sauces like Alfredo or Carbonara, as well as dishes with lots of cheese, such as manicotti or lasagna. Wise selections include tomato sauce (such as marinara or cacciatore) mushrooms or wine sauces (Marsala).

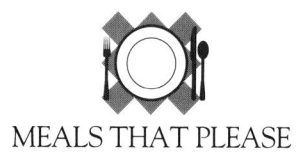

MEALS THAT PLEASE

485 CALORIES
3 stuffed mushrooms
Minestrone soup
Tossed salad with
1 Tbsp. reduced-calorie salad dressing
Italian bread stick
1 tsp. margarine

500 CALORIES
Chicken cacciatore
Side order of spaghetti marinara
Tossed salad with
1 Tbsp. reduced-calorie salad dressing

525 CALORIES
Spaghetti Marinara
1 slice Italian bread
Tossed salad with
1 Tbsp. reduced-calorie salad dressing

535 CALORIES
Veal piccata
Side order of pasta marinara
Italian garden salad with
1 Tbsp. reduced-calorie salad dressing

540 CALORIES
Pasta primavera (red sauce)
1 slice Italian bread
Tossed salad with
1 Tbsp. reduced-calorie salad dressing

550 CALORIES
Shrimp scampi
Baked potato/sour cream
Steamed broccoli
Italian garden salad with
1 Tbsp. reduced-calorie salad dressing

DINING OUT CHINESE STYLE

Chinese-style meals fit well into the nutrition guidelines for all Americans, as well as for people with diabetes. Vegetables are abundant. And foods can be low in fat and cholesterol.

Unfortunately, many Chinese dishes are high in sodium. They contain both MSG (monosodium glutamate) and high-sodium sauces, such as soy sauce and oyster sauce.

Chinese restaurants will often prepare to order. So, if sodium reduction is important to you, ask that MSG and soy sauce be eliminated in preparation. And don't be afraid to ask that less oil be used in food preparation. This will reduce fat content. Vegetables can be prepared steamed or with broth instead of oil.

Enjoy the variety, uniqueness, and change of taste that Chinese food offers your palate.

DINING TIPS

- Chinese restaurant menus are usually long, with many choices. So, know your meal plan and recognize portion sizes before you go. Portion control is important.
- A little of this and a little of that throughout dinner can really add up to a lot of food. If you are sharing dishes with friends, dish up your portion all at once. And don't go back for more.
- Choose dishes that are boiled, steamed, or lightly stir-fried. Avoid batter-fried and sweet and sour menu items.
- Egg rolls, fried shrimp, and fried won tons are deep-fried and therefore high in fat. Stay away from them.
- Pork-fried rice and beef-fried rice are high in fat. Stick with white rice. If you do order fried rice, order it vegetable-fried .
- If you are concerned about sodium content, remember that many Chinese soups are high in sodium.
- It's best to stay away from dishes that have nuts, such as almonds, cashews, or peanuts. They add extra calories.

MEALS THAT PLEASE

400 CALORIES
1 cup egg drop soup
2 cups chicken chow mein
2/3 cup rice
Tea

450 CALORIES
1 cup hot and sour soup
1/2 cup fried rice
2 oz. Chinese roast pork
1 cup stir-fry vegetables
1 fortune cookie
Tea

490 CALORIES
1 cup pepper steak
2/3 cup rice
Tea

495 CALORIES
1 1/2 cups beef chop suey
1/2 cup chow mein noodles
1/2 cup Chinese vegetables
1 fortune cookie
Tea

535 CALORIES
1 1/2 cups beef with vegetables
1/2 cup chow mein noodles
Tea

560 CALORIES
1 1/2 cups moo goo gai pan
2/3 cup rice
5 kumquats OR 2 fortune cookies
Tea

FAST FOOD

For most people, including those with diabetes, an occasional fast-food meal will not upset an otherwise healthy diet. When ordering fast food, the key is selection and serving size. You can limit calories, fat, and sodium by selecting wisely. Many fast-food restaurants help by offering salad bars, low-calorie salad dressings, soups, baked potatoes (easy on the toppings, please), broiled chicken sandwiches, diet soft drinks, low-fat milk, and frozen yogurts.

DINING TIPS

- Eat only at meal time. Try to balance a fast-food meal by carefully choosing your food for the rest of the day.
- Look for restaurants that have switched to unsaturated vegetable oil instead of animal/vegetable shortenings that contain beef tallow.
- Easy on the fried foods. Instead of French fries, have a baked potato filled with broccoli. If you eat French fries, order a small portion and complement your meal with a side salad. If broiled fish is offered, opt for it over fried. A grilled chicken sandwich is a better choice than the usual fried variety. If you do order fried, no extra crispy.
- Buy small. Words such as "jumbo," "giant," "extra large," or "deluxe" signal caution. Choose a single patty burger, not a double.
- Think healthy. Select a tossed salad and roll (skip the butter), or coleslaw and corn on the cob.
- Top smartly. Several fast-food chains offer baked potatoes. Enjoy one, but don't pile on bacon or sour cream. Top with broccoli and chives instead. As for pizza, top with mushrooms, green peppers, and onions.
- Skip the sauces. Replace the tartar sauce with lemon juice. Stay away from the sweet-and-sour, hot-mustard, and barbecue sauces. They add calories.

- Skip the mayonnaise. If a food item regularly comes with mayonnaise already on it, ask for one to be prepared without. You may have to wait a minute or two longer, but you'll be assured of a lower-fat item.
- Avoid milkshakes. They are high in fat and calories. Although some restaurants now offer low-fat milkshakes and frozen yogurt, they are still high in sugar. Choose diet colas or iced tea instead.

MEALS THAT PLEASE

350 CALORIES
Plain baked potato with
Chili topping
Diet cola

490 CALORIES
Quarter-pound hamburger with
Lettuce and tomato on a bun
Tossed salad with light vinaigrette dressing
Diet cola

500 CALORIES
Chicken breast fillet on bun
Coleslaw (1/2 cup)
Iced tea

550 CALORIES
Regular roast beef sandwich
Potato cakes
Diet cola

560 CALORIES
3 slices plain cheese pizza (16-inch diameter)

INDEX TO RECIPES

This index lists items by the menu in which they appear. B = breakfast; L = lunch; and D = dinner. For example, the entry, bay scallops parmesan, D21, indicates that that recipe is found in dinner 21.

Items underlined in the index are featured in menus, but no recipe is provided.

Page numbers refer to the dining out and snack sections of *Month of Meals 2*.

Month of Meals 1

The menus are simple, the recipes are easy, and the meals are tasty. The original *Month of Meals* has a whole new choice of breakfasts, lunches, and dinners (28 day's worth)—it's another monthly menu planner that does everything but put the food on your plate.

The cost is just $9.00 per copy for members or $10.00 per copy for nonmembers, plus shipping and handling.

To Order:

1. Write your name, address, and *Month of Meals #CMPMOM* on a piece of paper.
2. Tell us how many copies you want.
3. If you are an ADA member, write down your nine-digit ADA membership number (see the mailing label on *Diabetes Forecast*) to get your member discount.
4. If you live in Virginia, add 4.5% sales tax to the total.
5. Be sure to add shipping and handling using the chart below.
6. Send your order and a check or money order for *Month of Meals* to:
   American Diabetes Association
   1970 Chain Bridge Road
   McLean, VA 22109-0592

Shipping & Handling Chart
(calculate using the publications total)

up to $5.00	add $1.75
$5.01 - $10.00	add $3.00
$10.01 - $25.00	add $4.50
$25.01 - $50.00	add $5.50
over $50.00	add 10% of order

Make your check or money order payable to the American Diabetes Association. Allow 6-8 weeks for domestic delivery. Add $3.00 to shipping & handling for each additional "ship to" address. Add $15.00 to shipping & handling for air shipped orders outside the U.S. Prices subject to change without notice.

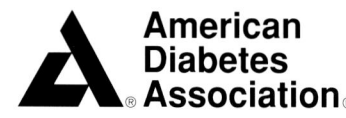